THE ENERGY SELF-DEFENSE SERIES - No. 8

ANNI & CARSTEN SENNOV

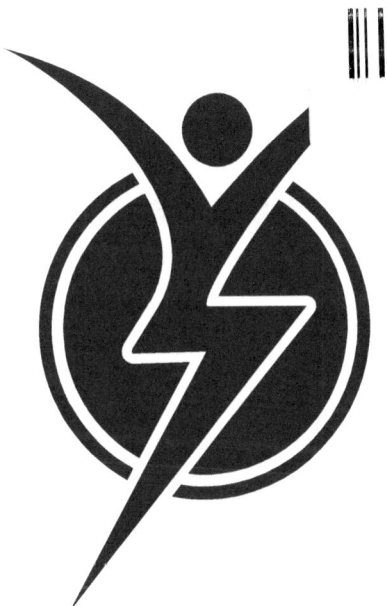

I0540514

ENERGY
SELF-DEFENSE
for
SICK PEOPLE
AND THEIR RELATIVES

good adventures publishing

Energy Self-Defense
for Sick People
and Their Relatives

©2018, Anni & Carsten Sennov and Good Adventures Publishing
First edition, first impression
Set with Cambria
Layout: Anni Sennov – www.sennovpartners.com
Cover design: Michael Bernth – www.monovoce.dk
Author photo: Aamod & Sophelia Korhonen – www.balanceisjoy.com

ISBN 978-87-7206-007-1

Contents

Notice

When reading this book, please be in a spirit of open-mindedness.

Although the authors and the publisher have made every effort to ensure the accuracy and completeness of information contained in this book, we assume no responsibility for errors, inaccuracies, omissions or any inconsistencies herein. Any offense caused to people, places or organizations is unintentional.

Readers should use their own judgment or consult a holistic medical expert or their personal physician for specific applications to their individual problems.

Intro

When we think about illness, we tend to think of an on-going disease which does not go away and may require daily medication, such as diabetes or thyroid disease. When we think of being sick, it may mean contracting the flu or just coming down with an everyday cold. With either situation, and along with injuries and accidents, this book will teach you some defining principles to help balance your body and mind, so you can fight for your health in a non-aggressive way.

As the authors of this book, we have both been seriously ill several times, and we also suffer from diseases that we are told can't be cured. Even so, that doesn't prevent us from living a wonderful, loving and rewarding life, although these health issues can sometimes be challenging.

We understand what you and your relatives are going through if you are suffering from a serious illness. We have both been in contact with many experts who are very skilled in traditional or Western medicine, as well as the alternative treatment world, to get the best treatments and help to be cured.

We have searched the Internet and read lots of books that share the latest research results, and discovered which herbs and roots are used to cure people with certain diseases all over the world. We have even read about curing ailments during the medieval times, and we have changed our lifestyle a couple of times to see if it would make a positive difference for us. We know how to reduce stress in everyday life, and we also know about many different types of health products, homeopathic remedies, nutrients and herbs that can help your physical body to get back into balance and recover from illness. However, that is not what we will focus on in this book.

It is important to note that we are not medical experts, and we suggest you consult with your medical advisor and/or your physician to give you personal advice on which medication or treatment is best for you.

We are instead experts in the field of Energy Self-Defense and we know how to protect and balance your personal energy and your body on an energetic level, and help you stand even stronger in yourself when dealing with physical or mental symptoms and challenges that you suffer from.

We also know a lot about spiritual energy and how to live a happy, balanced and stress-free life. When people get seriously ill, their life force is usually heavily compromised. Throughout this book you will learn how to recover and balance your body, mind and spirit in daily life, and especially when you become sick. As you begin learning about ways to use energy, you will hopefully get inspired to start thinking and living in a new and better way.

In this easy-to-read Energy Self-Defense guide for Sick People and Their Relatives, you will also get access to a lot of powerful and useful energy tools on how to protect, defend and balance your body and mind. In addition, we have personally tested all of these energy tools, and so have our partners and many of our clients. Anni's clairvoyant skills, spiritual knowledge, and ability to communicate with the invisible world on the other side of physical life, have lead us to write this very important book for the benefit of you and your relatives, where we share inside information about physical disease and physical pain, combined with spiritual knowledge.

Even if you have not experienced a serious illness, it is likely that you have a loved one who has. This book can be helpful to share with anyone who struggles with their own life force in the body on a daily basis.

So, if you are willing to "fight" for your life in a non-aggressive way with a focus on being positive, creating balance, and making room for the essence of life along with love and creativity – this is a "must read" book for you to recover and become alive again.

With love,

Anni & Carsten Sennov

Fight for your life
(1 mantra)

When you are sick you don't have to give up living a full life, so use this chapter to help you heal and balance your energy and ailments. It's actually possible for people to heal and balance their body energy, so the physical body can support them when they change direction and purpose in life, which is often the reason why people get seriously ill.

Imagine upgrading your personal energy to bring about a totally new life and a new healthy body.

It's absolutely amazing and miraculous to see how the life spark of a very sick person can suddenly be reignited because of personal will and the right treatment, and how this person's body energy and personal radiance are raised to a level that nobody would have ever expected.

Don't ever give up just because you have a diagnosis, even if you suffer from a life-threatening disease. Choose life and take extra good care of yourself, and accept the fact that you are right now about to change your life path, so the rest of your existing life may end up being very different from the life you had before you got sick.

Don't see yourself as being a sick and weak person, just because you must take medicine every day and maybe for the rest of your life. Instead, change your perspective on things and bless the medicine and treatments that you need to have, and try to accept the situation in the most balanced way you can.

This mantra can be very helpful for you to stay positive

and fight for your life. Say it out loud to yourself as often as you can:

"I now bless myself, my life, my body
and my daily medicine
and I neutralize all energies
in my life and my body
that don't match who I truly am deep inside.
I fill up and surround myself,
my life, my body and my medicine
with Divine positive energy
to create balance at all levels
in my life and my body."

Be open to change

Even if you don't feel ready to make radical changes in your life when you get seriously ill, you must be ready to change certain things, which may be the root cause of most diseases. The changes you make, however, don't have to happen in a negative way, even though disease is usually perceived as being negative. It can definitely be stressful and challenging physically, emotionally, and mentally when you are seriously ill. However, small changes can actually end up being very positive on many levels, even though it can be hard to believe when your body is out of sorts.

Always allow your body to recover and heal before you begin to transform your life dramatically. Don't ever make big decisions when you are very low on energy. Instead, take it one step at a time, where you allow your brain and heart to be able to adjust to the new life path that you are about to enter.

Change is hard for most people, and when you are sick it can seem even more difficult. You can compare acute illness and a serious disease to moving to a new house in a hurry, where you don't have time to pack and plan anything at all. The key to your new house and life path is found deep inside of yourself, but it's not yet visible. Therefore, you have to cope with everything in the new place as it is for now without being able to be organized and in control of things.

When you have managed to settle into your new place, which can take some time, you can go back and pick up your most precious belongings from your previous life in the place you lived before, if they are still there. Then you can start fresh, gathering all the pieces from your previous life that you want to bring into your new life and combine them with the current opportunities that you have in your new life, so you can start creating a whole new platform that will benefit you in the future.

Try to be as realistic as possible when you are in the process of arranging how your future life should be after you became ill, and don't be stubborn, refusing to change anything at all, because that will not benefit you in any way. Be happy that you are still alive and that there are people around you to support you and take good care of you, whether it's at home or in the hospital. There are so many things to be happy about in life that you may not have realized, because you were so focused on living your life in a certain way. Now all of a sudden there is a health issue which makes you change focus and opens up your mind to a new perspective and/or life path.

Take care of your personal energy, especially when you are sick

(1 mantra)

In general, it's very important for the health of your mind and body that you don't stress too much and that you try to eat healthy, drink lots of water, detox your body, get enough sleep, relax and meditate, and most important of all, rest and listen to your body and intuition. You know your own limitations, so don't expect or promise yourself to do something that you know deep inside is not possible for you to complete or achieve.

Stay positive and be happy for the things that you can do, and be realistic about who you are as a human – always be kind to yourself. Know that whatever decisions you make in life, you are the one responsible for the way that you live, and have to accept the consequences of your own lifestyle.

However, you not only have to take care of your body, but also your personal energy that radiates from your body. We call it Energy Self-Defense because we want you to learn how to defend your personal energy from being used, misused and/or stolen by others. It becomes even more important to do this when you are sick, and especially if there are others helping care for you.

Not everyone is as alert as they ought to be when it comes to listening to their body. They simply don't see the warning signs, or choose to ignore them. Most people usually get a forewarning when something is not working optimal in their body, and they may get a chance of changing things in their life before everything goes wrong. The problem, however, is that many people are actually their own worst enemies, and don't prioritize themselves enough. Therefore, they often end up becoming very sick as the result of their poor ability to take care of themselves, because they are so stubborn and unwilling to change the way they live.

Imagine if your breastfeeding child was allergic to dairy and the solution was for you to eliminate dairy in your diet. We bet you would do it in a heartbeat to help your growing child. When it comes to our own bodies, we often put ourselves on the backburner, when we know we should really do something proactive to help the situation.

Here is a very useful mantra that will help you to let go of stubbornness, and invite the flow of life into your everyday life and into your physical body:

"I now let go of all stubbornness
and all unwillingness to follow the flow of life,
and I become my own best friend,
who hereby invites
the eternal divine changeable flow of life
into my life and into my body."

Protect yourself and your body

There is a difference between being stubborn in a negative way, and being stubborn and persistent for the good of healing, i.e. adhering to a strict diet or routine to help your condition. Use your own determination and stubbornness to stay strong and open-minded, rather than sticking to your old ways of thinking.

If you hold on to your old ways of thinking and doing things that don't serve you anymore, then your mind and your body energy risk being reduced to a survival level where serious illness and disease belong. So instead, try a new approach and way of thinking if you want to heal up and get a new chance of living a balanced life in your existing body.

Are you too busy to think of yourself and take good care of your body, or are you more concerned about taking care of others and forget to take care of yourself? It's imperative to focus on your own body and health, because if you don't, your body will likely force you to do it, which will usually happen in a way that you don't want.

Wake up and start focusing on your physical body, which is the most visible and dense part of you, and the current home of your spirit and personal energy. Be honest with yourself: what is the reason why you don't take good care of your physical body?

If you have a very high-flying spiritual energy, your excuse may be that you don't find life on Planet Earth very intelligent and exciting.

If you are very grounded and somewhat heavy in your physical energy and appearance, you are likely to be focused on how you can benefit from life, and what you can eat, buy and own, etc. Therefore, you are not so concerned about others. You mainly focus on your own family or group of friends and companions, your so-called tribe, and how to survive, and your main excuse for not listening to your own body and its needs is that you are too busy.

If you belong to the very big group of people who trust commercials and believe for example that diet food and diet drinks are actually okay for you because there is artificial sugar in them instead of "real sugar", you are not excused at all for not knowing better. If you watch television and search the Internet a lot, you have the tools to get all the information you need to change your priorities in life. It may take time to gather information about how to take good care of yourself and what to eat, etc. After gaining knowledge from various sources, your inner voice will be activated and will allow you to start focusing on the types of things you can start doing to take better care of yourself.

It may sound strange to you that a person can actually protect their own body, using something other than a weapon. However, you can easily protect your body from being sick by eating healthy, getting physical exercise on a daily basis, dancing, and doing other activities to help your body feel better and be stronger.

They say laughter is the best medicine! When you laugh your body begins to vibrate at a much higher frequency, which is also the case when you practice yoga and meditate. When you balance and protect your body by eating heathy and doing physical exercises on a daily basis, your body will be a happier home for your spirit – which is **the real you** – allowing you to live a more satisfied life with less challenges and symptoms in your body.

Treat your body right, and it will also treat you right!!!

By protecting your physical body, you automatically protect yourself, and if you have problems protecting yourself, you should use the Energy Self-Defense mantras and exercises that we share in this book. They will make you feel better, so you can take even better care of your body, which is an essential part of you being a human. Without your body, there is no **you** in the physical world, which will hopefully motivate you to take extra good care of **the whole you**, now that you are here and alive and spending time together with your loved ones.

Always appreciate life and what it has to offer, and if you are not satisfied with how things are, then try to change them by taking positive action and visualizing how you want things to be.

Protect yourself even when others are caring for you
(3 mantras)

When you are sick and very low on energy, you often need treatment or advice from your medical doctor or therapist. As you are being treated by health professionals, it's extremely important that you pull all your rightful energy back from these people, places and situations when you leave, even if you are supposed to get better when you go there. Let us explain why.

The fact is that many people go to the ER and the clinic every day to get help and advice because they are seriously ill and don't feel well. They're typically not cured when they leave the hospital, because they need medication or a certain type of treatment to be cured. So, while they are waiting for help, they usually don't surround themselves with positive energy, because they are in pain or tired, and feeling terrible, not to mention they are also near other patients who are suffering as well and not being very positive either.

Many people have to wait for long hours and maybe even days or weeks for their results before the doctor tells them which medicine and treatment they need in order to get well. So usually there is a certain amount of anxiety or suppressed and sad energy in places where people go to be cured.

Think of a relaxing day spa or places which have treatments that are good for you, and where the energy is much higher, more positive, and people feel hope and surround themselves with happiness. It is very important for those who are sick, as well as for their relatives and the staff working at hospitals and clinics, to pull all of their own individual energy back and bring it with them when they leave. Otherwise they risk going home with an energy that is not their own, and they will respond to that energy as if it was their own, which can make them feel worse than they usually do.

Here are several mantras that will help you protect your energy, pull back your own energy from others, and bless the spaces you are receiving treatment in:

> *"I now pull all my rightful energy*
> *back to myself*
> *from the places and situations I've been in,*
> *and from the people I've been together with*
> *– in a cleansed form –*
> *and I send all the rightful energy*
> *of these places, situations and people*
> *out of my own energy field*
> *and return it to where it came from."*

If you feel that it is very hard for you to sit and wait for a long time in a place with sick people around you, or you feel intruded upon or affected by the things that are happening around you, we recommend that you repeat the following mantra as many times as you like to neutralize the energy around you:

> *"I now bless all the people around me*
> *as well as the place and situation I'm in,*
> *and I neutralize the energies between us*
> *with Divine and positive energy."*

You can also say this mantra where you focus on creating good energy within yourself:

*"I now embrace myself
in a pure white light/energy
to dissolve and neutralize all negative energies
around me and create balance."*

Love and embrace your body and life
(1 mantra)

Always honor and bless your body and love and embrace it, because it is your earthly home in a totally different way than the place you live in. You can always move out of the place you live in, but you can't move out of your body, so you must take good care of it.

When combined with the mental and spiritual energy tools that we share with you in this book, your body is the strongest earthly energy tool you have. This is because your body is filled with physical materialization power, which all people need to be able to act out things in life and succeed. The main concern is whether or not your body is in the right energy frequency to match who you really are deep inside.

If not, you might be placed in the danger zone outside of your personal "energy comfort zone" where you don't feel truly at home in your own body, and then you are more likely than others to get sick or even become seriously ill.

It's necessary for you to be in sync with your physical body at all levels to avoid becoming sick.

A good place to start loving and embracing yourself is to bless your life, especially if you are not satisfied with how things currently are. Everything you surround yourself with and everything you do is a part of you and what you radiate into the world, so if you don't like the current state of things, you must start making changes from a place deep inside of yourself. This will help you to radiate a happier, more balanced and calm energy to the surrounding world, instead of radiating the underlying stress that you feel in your body every day from living in a way which is out of sync with your body.

When you bless yourself, your life and your body, you thereby start attracting new possibilities into your life that match the inner you and help you to become in sync with your body. The following mantra will help you to create a better energy foundation for your body, so it will better match who you really are deep inside:

"I now bless myself, my life and my body,
and neutralize all energies
in my life and my body
that don't match who I truly am deep inside.
I fill up my life and my body
with Divine positive energy
to create balance at all levels
in my life and in my body."

Be in charge of your own life and health

(2 mantras)

Medical doctors and therapists are the experts in medicine and treatments, but they are not experts in how to live **your** life. Therefore, we recommend that you get all the help and the expertise from them that you can, but remember that you are the one who knows deep inside what is best for you. So, unless you suffer from a mental disease where you are unable to make reasonable decisions that benefit yourself, you should always ask your own body, as well as other experts and God for a second opinion. Then you will feel more confident and in charge of making your own decisions based on all the knowledge you gather from these various sources.

It's also important to decide which relatives and friends you should listen to and get support and good advice from. Not everyone is qualified for that role. Therefore, you must decide which people should be allowed to be close to you when you are sick, and how much information you'll want to share with them about your current situation.

Depending on the type of illness and severity of your situation, some people will feel inclined to share your health story with others, unbeknownst to you. Perhaps they are in shock, or it's too emotional for them to deal with. Most certainly, they will talk about you and your disease with anyone who wants to listen to them, while they try to digest and deal with your situation. Every time they talk with others, they will feel relieved inside, which will continue on until the day they can deal with the whole situation in a more balanced way. So, expect your personal story to be spread in different circles, until these people have emptied their emotional containers.

As you can imagine, there will most certainly be lots of stress and unbalanced energy around you that belongs to other people who are trying to process your situation. Therefore, it's extremely important that you sort your energies on a daily basis.

If you surround yourself with people who feel pity or feel sorry for you because you are sick, then return the pity to sender. It's okay if they feel compassion for you, as this emotion is loaded with a much more positive energy than the feeling of pity.

If people around you become afraid or even get scared because your disease reminds them of their own vulnerability in life, then you should also return the energy to sender, no matter if they send you positive or negative energy. People who are afraid to die or get seriously ill will usually be extra concerned and worried when they think of you. They will try not to think of you, or they will feel scared when they think of you, and there is generally nothing positive for you to get from these people, even if they are kind people. Therefore, you should immediately return their energy back to them.

Being in charge of your own life and your own energy also means returning people's energy back to them. It can be done many times a day. Just repeat the following mantra as often as you like:

"I now pull all my rightful energy
back to myself from 'X'
– in a cleansed form –
and I send all the rightful energy of 'X'
out of my own energy field and body
and return it to him/her/them."

Maybe it's time for you to also let go of the past, and reflect to gain understanding, so you can leave everything that happened behind you.

Do your best to live in the present and don't allow yourself to be haunted by your past, because there is nothing you can do to undo your previous actions. You can however try to change the energy in and around the things and situations that you are not satisfied with by forgiving, sorting and separating your energy from everybody in your past, whether they were good or bad people. The essence of this exercise is that it will set you free on an energetic level and give you peace of mind, so that you are no longer energetically influenced by things that happened a long time ago.

You can let go of your past by repeating this mantra frequently throughout the day:

"I now forgive myself and 'X'
and everybody else
for what happened in my past,
and I forgive myself,
because I have kept the tensions,
sadness, aggression and frustration in me
that was created in my past.
I now let go of all negative things
that happened in my past
and create space for new positive

experiences and energies in my life,
and I send the rightful energy of 'X'
and everybody else in my past
out of my own energy field and body
and return it to them."

When you use this mantra to forgive and let go of the past, all of your rightful energy that has previously been stuck in the past will automatically be returned to you.

Hate can make you very sick
(1 mantra)

Did you know that you can actually get very sick if you feel haunted by your past, and if you think about other people too much, especially if you think about people who make you feel angry or sad? If the feelings of anger, frustration and sadness take control of your mind and you think about or focus on negative people and situations quite often, then that very negative energy will automatically find its way into your body, and you risk getting sick.

Negative energy is like poison. Try and focus on the good things in life and pay less attention to negative things. This, however, doesn't mean that you should ignore negative energy completely. Instead, you should protect your own energy by sending negativity back to where it came from, and by being honest with yourself. If something doesn't feel right for you, then always say "NO" so you don't trespass your own boundaries and risk getting angry later on.

What you may not know is that energy can always be used by the receiver, no matter if it is positive or negative. When you get angry at other people and think about them a lot, they can actually use your energy to succeed just as well as if you're supporting them with positive energy. It all depends on their personality.

If they are kind and sensitive people, you may not have problems with them at all. In this case you won't need to protect your own energy. Such relationships are usually very balanced and rewarding for both parties.

If they are aggressive, negative and greedy people, they will usually steal and digest the energy that you send out no matter if it is positive or negative. So always pull back your outstanding energy when you are together with such people, as they don't share energy. They take it all for themselves so even if it sounds tempting, don't send them lots of negative energy, because then they will become even more nasty.

When you use the following mantra to claim your rightful energy and get it back from people you dislike or even hate, and then return their respective energies back to them as well, you will often feel how the positive energy starts to flow in your veins. The more you repeat this mantra, the more you will get an increase in positive energy, and a better flow of energy within your physical body. This is because hate has a very strong impact on the densest part of your energy (which is your physical body), so when the hate and negativity leave your body, you will almost feel reborn:

"I now pull all my rightful energy back to myself
from all people who I dislike and hate
– in a cleansed form –
and I send all their rightful energy
out of my own energy field and body
and return it to them."

Where did your energy go?
And how to get it back
(6 mantras)

We have all had days where we feel drained and lack energy. However, if you are truly not healthy and happy, then you should go and find your missing energy, because apparently you left it somewhere outside of your own body, or someone has unrightfully taken it from you.

You can be sick for a variety of reasons, which we will not elaborate on here. Instead we will share with you how to find your missing energy:

1)

First have a look around you to see if other people you know have suddenly become more healthy and happy at the same time that you started to feel worse.

They may be happy as a result of their own effort, so don't judge them just because they are happy and feel good. However, if you feel that they have somehow benefitted from your energy without you being aware of it, it's time for you to get your lost energy back.

2)

Now pull all your rightful energy back from the relevant people. Draw your energy through a cleansing filter, so it's only your own energy that is returned to you, and not the energy of others:

*"I now pull all my rightful energy
back to myself from 'X'
– in a cleansed form –
and I send all the rightful energy of 'X'
out of my own energy field and body
and return it to him/her/them."*

3)

Soon you will start to feel a positive change in yourself. If your energy has been in other people's bodies and energy systems for a very long time, they most certainly think it is their own energy, and it may take some time to get your energy back from them.

When you get your energy back, it is extremely important that you clean the energy. Remember that it has been and still might be integrated in another person's energy field, and you only want your own energy back.

4)

If you don't know who has taken your energy you should simply replace 'X' with 'everybody' and don't focus on getting your energy back from any specific person(s).

5)

It's very important that you reclaim your own rightful power and energy and get rid of other people's energy, which can be done by sorting your energies and dissolving all bad energies between you and others, etc. Practice the following 5 steps, and repeat the mantras as often as you wish. It will help you to clean up and balance all of your relationships, and hopefully make you feel stronger in your personal energy and in your body.

Step 1: Sort your energies

Start by sorting your energies so that you get your rightful energy back from all the people, places and situations that bother you and make you angry, sad or sick. Repeat this energy sorting mantra as often as you like:

"I now pull all my rightful energy back to myself
from all the people, places and situations
that bother me and make me angry, sad and sick
– in a cleansed form –
and I send all their rightful energy
out of my own energy field and body
and return it to them."

Step 2: Dissolve all bad energies between you and others

Now visualize that you embrace yourself and all the people, places and situations that make you angry, sad or sick with white light/energy, to neutralize all negative energies that have ever existed between you:

"I now embrace myself
and all the people, places and situations
that make me angry, sad and sick
in a pure white light/energy
to dissolve all bad energies between us."

Step 3: Forgive yourself

The most important thing is for you to forgive yourself for what happened and let go of the past, which will happen when you use this mantra:

"I now forgive myself
and all the people, places and situations
that make me angry, sad and sick
for what happened.
I now let go of all that happened
and create space for new positive
experiences and energies in my life."

Step 4: Set boundaries

If the people, places and situations continue to anger you
or get on your nerves, you can separate your energies from
them by using this mantra:

"I now place a thick wall
of blue boundary-setting energy
between me
and all the people, places and situations
that make me angry, sad and sick
to separate our energies
and to keep them and their energy
away from me."

Step 5: Did others spread out your energy?

If you have a feeling or know that the people that make you
angry, sad or sick have spread out **your energy** to others in
their network, or if others have benefited from the energy
that they have taken from you, you should pull back all of
your energy from those people.

Similarly, if you have a strong feeling that other people
whom you don't know have benefited from the energy that

you shared in certain places and situations, you should also pull back all of your energy from them.

Your energy is your rightful energy, and it should always be around you and not around others – no matter who they are or how much you love them. Say the following energy-sorting mantra to influence people who have taken energy from you, their network and anyone they have influenced by using your energy:

"I now pull all my rightful energy back to myself
from all the people, places and situations
that make me angry, sad and sick
and from their network or from whomever
they shared my energy with
– in a cleansed form –
and I send all the rightful energy of
all the people, places and situations
that make me angry, sad and sick
out of my own energy field and body
and return it to them."

What makes you happy
may make you healthy

It's always good to pay attention to and appreciate the small signs of progress when you are sick. It gives you hope, which is loaded with positive energy that can activate faster healing of your body and mind.

If you're not a fan of taking prescription medicine, then try to create a lot of good energy around your daily medicine procedure and make it a happy and positive experience. Sit in a beautiful place and enjoy the morning sun or surround yourself with things that make you happy. Enjoy your favorite dish while taking your medicine, or listen to your favorite song. Simply find out what makes you happy and combine it with the things that you are not so thrilled about, like taking your medicine, to make you feel better.

Always be kind to yourself and your body and don't accept things that are not good for you. Remember to take good care of your body and eat and sleep well, rest when you need it, go for a walk to exercise your body even if you are sick and tired, surround yourself with good energy and positive vibes, and spend time with kind and supportive people.

Never accept sleeping on a couch that is not comfortable, or sleeping or staying in a room with no possibility of opening the windows to get fresh air. Nature is your best friend and your body will recover much faster when you spend time outdoors. When you breathe deeply you oxygenate your body. That is why ozone therapy has become so popular, because your body needs oxygen to give life to and nourish the cells.

Try and surround yourself with positive energy before you go to bed, so your body and brain can relax and be loaded with balanced energy during the night. As you can imagine, it is not recommended that you watch violent movies or disturbing documentaries before you go to sleep, because the violent energy risks activating the survival energy in you, and not the balanced energy that your body needs to recover and reload itself while you sleep.

Maybe you feel that there are way too many requirements to follow if you want to live a good and healthy life, and that you must invest a lot of time, effort, and money to be able to feel good. You may even think that it's not worth it and that you don't want to limit yourself in any way. If you don't listen to what your body wants, and you don't give it what it needs, you may end up becoming seriously ill because you don't want to eat healthy or quit smoking, etc.

On one hand, if it makes you happy to eat unhealthy food and smoke cigarettes every day, you are already doing what makes you feel happy, and feeling happy inside may make you live longer. However, if what makes you happy is not good for your body, you will one day have to accept the fact that changes are needed if you want to live a LONG and happy life, and not just a happy life.

It's very interesting to observe people who are told that they will not survive for much longer if they don't change their lifestyle, and see how they suddenly start to love everything that is good for their body. It's like a new life-oriented and caring mindset is suddenly being activated in their energy system that makes them listen to what their body wants, because if they don't, they will soon become sicker and then it will become harder for them to recover.

So, what makes you happy can suddenly change from one

minute to the next depending on how sick you are and how bad you feel in your body, which is why you should always listen to your body.

When it's time to recover

Once you have broken the disease curve and it's time to recover, it's important that you don't press yourself too hard. Don't have super high expectations for yourself and your body, because if you get stressed or push your body beyond its limits, your body will soon change from being stressed, to becoming a body in pain. Therefore, remember to give yourself time.

The recovery period can be compared to a period where you prepare to be more kind to yourself and learn to listen to the signals coming from your body. Soon you will be able to better understand your own body and meet its needs, and you will end up becoming an expert in taking good care of yourself by using the Energy Self-Defense tools, and living your life to the fullest in a balanced way.

When your body has fully recovered, and you have learned everything there is to know about how to take care of yourself and your body, you can decide for yourself which skills and knowledge you'll want to implement as part of your future life.

You are never going to forget how you felt when you were seriously ill, so you will never be the same person as you were before you got sick. Hopefully the way you treat yourself will also be changed for the better.

How can you as a relative help a sick person?

(2 mantras)

As a relative of a very sick person, you often suffer as much as the sick person, but in a different way. You see and feel everything from the outside, and often there is nothing you can do to make the person feel better other than being present, and doing your best to help the sick person feel comfortable.

It's not your own body and energy that needs healing, but there are actually plenty of things you can do to help the sick person feel better. All you have to do is ask the sick person for permission to use all the Energy Self-Defense tools mentioned in this book to help him/her.

If you don't get permission, you are certainly not allowed to do anything on behalf of the sick person. Please note that you are never allowed to trespass another person's boundaries, not even if they are physically sick. Only when they are mentally sick and you are their guardian, then can you assist.

As a relative, one of the worst things you can do to a seriously ill person who you love, is to feel pity and sorry for them. Instead, feel compassion and be supportive, and try to be good spirited and as happy as you possibly can be whenever you are near them. Even though they know they are very sick and weak, the feeling of pity and weakness doesn't do any good for them. It's very demotivating to feel weak and know that other people feel pity whenever they hear about your situation. Any progress is then automatically diminished, and it makes it much harder for the sick person's mind to overcome physical obstacles and challenges, especially when it's time to rehabilitate and get back to life. Try to be as positive as possible and don't comment on things if you don't have anything positive to say.

If it is hard for you to be near your sick relative and to see how the life is flowing out of them, try not to feel sorry for yourself. If you fall into that very deep hole, it can take an extremely long time for you to crawl back out again. Of course, it's okay that you feel sad and depressed, but self-pity can be compared to having depression, and you should never allow yourself to be influenced by the whole situation in that way. We recommend that you use the following mantras to keep your personal energy in balance whenever you are together with the sick person, and when you think of him/her when you are not together:

"I now embrace myself
and my relationship to the sick person
in pink love energy
to activate and radiate love
in our relationship and between us,
so we will both feel better
and I will keep my inner balance
whenever I'm together with,
or think of the sick person."

and

"I now embrace myself,
the sick person, and our relationship
in a pure white light/energy
to dissolve all bad energies around us
and our relationship,
and to keep away the feeling of self-pity
from my energy field and my body."

If you want to help the sick person by using your own energy, it can be done by thinking about him/her a lot and sending lots of love and positive thoughts. Even though you might not be able to cure him/her, you can perhaps help them feel better.

Note that you should always pull back your own energy – you decide when – since you need the energy yourself. If they suddenly begin to feel better, you should consider pulling back your energy immediately. If this is not done, the sick person will have your energy available for as long as you allow them to.

Taking back your energy is important to do even if it makes the sick person appear to get sicker as a result. Maybe you are afraid of hurting them by taking back your energy, but ultimately that's what's best for everyone, since the sick person cannot expect to live long on your energy. He/she will have to survive and learn to live their life based on their own energy – not yours.

If you are worried that the sick person will not survive, and you want to help, we warmly recommend that you repeat the two mantras mentioned earlier in this chapter. They represent all the best you can do to help others without weakening your own energy.

The importance of having a strong aura in the healing process

As a clairvoyant advisor and the founder of the healing modality called AuraTransformation™, Anni knows the importance of having a strong aura to protect your physical body.

An aura is a kind of energetic shield and protection that envelops your body, and among other things, it is meant to protect your body from outside energies and help keep your own energies to yourself. While most people cannot see auras, it is definitely something they can sense, as an aura can also send out a "vibe" about how a person is feeling for example.

The aura also has an intelligence of its own. If you are very weak and almost about to die, your aura will do its best to adapt to your current life situation and automatically start becoming weaker, so that it doesn't counteract your underlying or unconscious desire to die.

After being involved in a serious accident or after undergoing a major surgery, the aura is usually flapping around the body, unable to find its balance. This is because it has been completely stressed out by all the different signals that are sent from the body during the accident/surgery. As a result, most people feel very sensitive and unprotected after an accident/major surgery, and have a hard time healing.

To put it simply, the aura doesn't always know if a person is supposed to survive or die during an accident/surgery. If the aura is not brought into balance after an accident/major surgery, the person will usually feel dizzy for a long time and the aura and body will not be in sync with each other.

In fact, they will often try to move in different directions energy-wise, which means that they will both constantly be switching between searching for life and searching for death. This is not necessarily because the person wants to die, but because the aura and body intelligences don't know what else to do.

Back in the "old days" people actually died when they lost their aura in an accident, but today most people can easily survive the loss of their aura. The result of this however is that they get overly sensitive or very sick.

For example, in the summer of 2010 Anni was contacted by an 82 year old woman, who knew deep in her heart that Anni would be able to help a mutual friend, who at that time was 85 years old and had been violently struck by a car. The mutual friend was Anni's old anatomy teacher, who was a very powerful and engaging woman who always helped others. She had been in the hospital for a while and was not fully conscious, and she had black bruises all over the body from the severe accident.

Nobody aside from the family was allowed to visit her, and they all thought it was time to say their goodbyes. However, when her son asked her if she wanted Anni to help her get her energy and strength back, she smiled without opening her eyes. The next day Anni went to the hospital to help her gather her aura around her body, and guess what happened?

After two hours the patient was able to sit up in the hospital bed and started speaking slowly, and suddenly she became very hungry and more alive in her physical body. After three hours she commented on how the nurse did her job, and after two days she was transferred to a rehabilitation center where she stayed for a few months, because she was not yet strong enough to take care of herself in everyday life.

This amazing woman never quite got the balance back in her legs, but she lived for another six years and continued to help other people in the way she did before the accident.

In another example, in 2014 our 13 year old daughter went through a major surgery where two surgeons worked simultaneously on her back for seven hours. She was very weak after the surgery, so we placed high-frequency patches on several areas of her body, and she managed to leave the hospital with less pain than expected two days before her scheduled discharge. When we got home, Anni suddenly discovered that our daughter's aura was not as big and strong as it used to be, or as it was supposed to be. So Anni adjusted and balanced her aura so it could unfold again in full size, and thereafter our daughter became more mobile, recovered faster physically, and in no time was back in school.

It turned out that our daughter had been under anesthesia for so many hours that her aura had almost collapsed, and it thought that it didn't need to ever unfold again. During anesthesia, or you could say during this unconscious state, her body didn't send out any signals to the aura confirming that she was still alive and needed protection around her body, which is what the aura gives you.

In 1996, Anni founded and established AuraTransforma-tion™ in Denmark, which is now widespread throughout the world. As you might imagine, the importance of having a strong aura is not new to Anni. These two incidents really opened our eyes and made us both understand the bigger role that the aura plays in all people's lives, especially when it comes to recovery and regaining the balance and life force in the body after being seriously ill. When you have a strong aura, it is much easier for you to choose life rather than death, and your healing process will automatically happen at a much faster pace.

AuraTransformation™ is a permanent expansion of your personal consciousness and a powerful upgrade to your aura structure, which creates synergy between your charisma, drive, intuition and physical actions. The main purpose of having an AuraTransformation™ is to transform and upgrade your personal energy, radiance and human protection so that you will always attract balance in your personal life for the benefit of yourself and those around you. It helps your inner truth to come forward, and then you can no longer lie to yourself or close down your inner senses. You simply follow your inner truth no matter where it leads you in your physical life.

It is important to note that AuraTransformation™ is *not* a cure, but a healing modality that strengthens your aura and the energetic protection around your body, so you can easily connect with your own spirit.

Visit **www.auratransformation.com** to learn more.

Useful energy tools
(16 mantras)

In this chapter we have added all the mantras mentioned within this book, so you can get a good overview of which mantras to use in different situations. It is important that you read the whole book to get a good understanding of how, why and when to use each mantra.

TIP!

Take a picture of your favorite mantras on your phone, to always keep them with you when you need them.

Bless yourself and your daily medicine:

> *"I now bless myself, my life, my body*
> *and my daily medicine*
> *and I neutralize all energies*
> *in my life and my body*
> *that don't match who I truly am deep inside.*
> *I fill up and surround myself,*
> *my life, my body and my medicine*
> *with Divine positive energy*
> *to create balance at all levels*
> *in my life and my body."*

Let go of your stubbornness and invite the flow into your life:

> *"I now let go of all stubbornness*
> *and all unwillingness to follow the flow of life,*
> *and I become my own best friend,*

who hereby invites
the eternal divine changeable flow of life
into my life and into my body."

Take your energy back from places where people get treatment:

"I now pull all my rightful energy
back to myself
from the places and situations I've been in,
and from the people I've been together with
– in a cleansed form –
and I send all the rightful energy
of these places, situations and people
out of my own energy field
and return it to where it came from."

Neutralize the energy around you in places where you wait for treatment:

"I now bless all the people around me
as well as the place and situation I'm in,
and I neutralize the energies between us
with Divine and positive energy."

Create good energy in yourself when you wait for treatment:

"I now embrace myself
in a pure white light/energy
to dissolve and neutralize all negative energies
around me and create balance."

Help your body match who you truly are deep inside:

"I now bless myself, my life and my body,
and neutralize all energies
in my life and my body
that don't match who I truly am deep inside.
I fill up my life and my body
with Divine positive energy
to create balance at all levels
in my life and in my body."

Sort your energies:

"I now pull all my rightful energy
back to myself from 'X'
– in a cleansed form –
and I send all the rightful energy of 'X'
out of my own energy field and body
and return it to him/her/them."

and

"I now pull all my rightful energy back to myself
from all the people, places and situations
that bother me and make me angry, sad and sick
– in a cleansed form –
and I send all their rightful energy
out of my own energy field and body
and return it to them."

Let go of your past:

"I now forgive myself and 'X'
and everybody else

for what happened in my past,
and I forgive myself,
because I have kept the tensions,
sadness, aggression and frustration in me
that was created in my past.
I now let go of all negative things
that happened in my past
and create space for new positive
experiences and energies in my life,
and I send the rightful energy of 'X'
and everybody else in my past
out of my own energy field and body
and return it to them."

Get your energy back from people you don't like:

"I now pull all my rightful energy back to myself
from all people who I dislike and hate
– in a cleansed form –
and I send all their rightful energy
out of my own energy field and body
and return it to them."

Dissolve all bad energies between you and others:

"I now embrace myself
and all the people, places and situations
that make me angry, sad and sick
in a pure white light/energy
to dissolve all bad energies between us."

Forgive yourself:

"I now forgive myself
and all the people, places and situations
that make me angry, sad and sick
for what happened.
I now let go of all that happened
and create space for new positive
experiences and energies in my life."

Set boundaries:

"I now place a thick wall
of blue boundary-setting energy
between me
and all the people, places and situations
that make me angry, sad and sick
to separate our energies
and to keep them and their energy
away from me."

Get your energy back from those who
you have shared your energy with:

"I now pull all my rightful energy back to myself
from all the people, places and situations
that make me angry, sad and sick
and from their network or from whomever
they shared my energy with
– in a cleansed form –
and I send all the rightful energy of
all the people, places and situations
that make me angry, sad and sick
out of my own energy field and body
and return it to them."

Mantras for relatives:

"I now embrace myself
and my relationship to the sick person
in pink love energy
to activate and radiate love
in our relationship and between us,
so we will both feel better
and I will keep my inner balance
whenever I'm together with,
or think of the sick person."

and

"I now embrace myself,
the sick person, and our relationship
in a pure white light/energy
to dissolve all bad energies around us
and our relationship,
and to keep away the feeling of self-pity
from my energy field and my body."

Thank you for reading

If you want to know more about how to protect and defend your personal energy in your life, please visit our website:

www.energyselfdefense.com

Here you will find information about our collection of helpful energy guides in our Energy Self-Defense series. We suggest that you begin with *"Energy Self-Defense for Women"* and/or *"Energy Self-Defense for Men"*, where you will benefit from advice on how to achieve a more balanced life on a personal level. You can also participate in our Energy Self-Defense online courses.

To learn more about the authors, please feel free to visit our other websites:

www.sennovpartners.com

www.annisennov.com

www.carstensennov.com

We hope that you are pleased with what you have learned from reading this Energy Self-Defense guide, and that you are going to use the Mantras often, and integrate them into your daily routine.

Please tell your family, friends, colleagues and neighbors about our Energy Self-Defense series, so that we can hopefully work collectively to make this a better world to live in for everyone.

A good way to spread the word about how to take care of your own energy, is by giving the pocket-sized *"The Little Energy Guide 1"* to those you love and care about.

Finally, you can spread good energy by rating and commenting on this book at the website where you bought it, as well as on Anni Sennov's author page at **Goodreads.com**.

We know how much it means to everyone to have good health, so if you know of anyone who is seriously ill, or if you know people who are related to someone struggling with a serious illness, you can help them by recommending them to read this energy guide.

We wish you and your loved one(s) a quick and full recovery, and a long, happy and healthy life.

Anni & Carsten Sennov